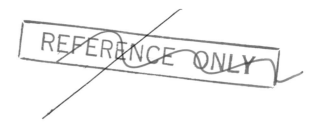

A Colour Atlas of
Ear Disease

A Colour Atlas of
Ear Disease

Richard A. Chole
M.D., Ph.D.

Associate Professor
Department of Otorhinolaryngology
School of Medicine
University of California
Davis, California

Wolfe Medical Publications Ltd

Copyright © R. A. Chole, 1982
Published by Wolfe Medical Publications Ltd, 1982
Printed by Royal Smeets Offset b.v., Weert, Netherlands

ISBN 0 7234 0776 2

This book is one of the titles in the series of
Wolfe Medical Atlases, a series which brings
together probably the world's largest systematic
published collection of diagnostic colour
photographs.
For a full list of Atlases in the series, plus
forthcoming titles and details of our surgical,
dental and veterinary Atlases, please write to
Wolfe Medical Publications Ltd, Wolfe House,
3 Conway Street, London W1P 6HE

Contents

Dedicated to my children,
Joey, Tim, Katy and Melinda,
who were the willing subjects of
many of the photographs in this atlas.

Introduction

Otoscopy and the physical diagnosis of otologic disease remain one of the most difficult portions of the physical examination for clinicians. A physician-in-training may only have opportunity to see a fraction of the otologic diseases that he may encounter as a practitioner. In many cases, when a pathological condition is seen, it is not recognized because of lack of prior experience with that disease entity. In addition, the anatomy of the external auditory canal precludes simple otoscopic techniques.

While the human tympanic membrane is approximately 9mm in diameter, the external auditory canal, even in the adult, is rarely larger than 5-6mm. Therefore, only a small portion of the tympanic membrane can be seen by direct optical techniques. The examiner must position a conventional otoscope toward the various quadrants of the tympanic membrane in order to see the entire structure. The anterior sulcus of the tympanic membrane and the external auditory canal is usually obscured by the anterior canal wall, which represents a prominence due to the underlying glenoid fossa. Even with the aid of the operating microscope, only small portions of the tympanic membrane can be seen at any one time (*see* Figure **1**).

Most previous attempts to photograph the tympanic membrane have been thwarted by the aforementioned anatomical facts. Successful photographs have been obtained therefore only in patients with large external auditory canals, and we have had to satisfy ourselves with photographs of the central portion of the tympanic membrane. The recent introduction of the Hopkins* rod lens system has allowed photography of the entire tympanic membrane by advancing a narrow rod lens past the narrow isthmus of the external auditory canal and obtaining a wide angle photograph of the drumhead from that viewpoint (*see* Figure **2**). When viewed through this optical system, one can usually see the entire drumhead, including the tympanic annulus in all quadrants. In rare cases, a very prominent anterior wall still precludes visualization of that area. Because of the large depth of field of this optical system, all areas of the canal and tympanic membrane appear to be in focus.

The photographs used in this atlas were obtained by adapting the otologic telescope (Karl Storz 1218A), which is 2.7mm in diameter, to a 35mm single lens reflex camera, using a 135mm focal length lens. A high-intensity, xenon electronic flash tube was placed adjacent to the fibre optic bundle of the telescope for illumination during photography. High Speed (ASA 400) colour transparency film was used throughout. The image produced by this system was 24mm in diameter, which fills a conventional 35mm slide. The camera and lighting system are self contained and portable (Figure **3**), so that the camera could be quickly transported to other hospitals or clinics when interesting or unusual otoscopic findings were present.

The purpose of this atlas is to familiarise the physician with the physical diagnosis of the tympanic membrane and its diseases. An attempt has been made to gather a large number of pathological conditions, as well as to include several examples of each. Histological and radiographic material is included for the purpose of clarifying physical findings.

*Karl Storz Endoscopy

1

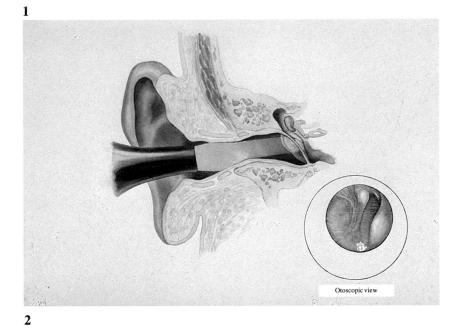

Otoscopic view

2

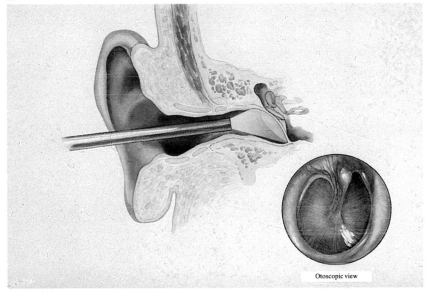

Otoscopic view

3

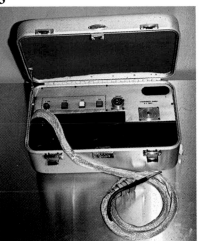

Normal tympanic membrane

4 Normal right tympanic membrane The normal tympanic membrane is translucent and takes on the reddish colour of the underlying middle ear mucosa. It is a conical structure which is approximately 9 millimeters in diameter. It is divided into a small upper pars flaccida (1) and a lower pars tensa (2). The short process of the malleus (3) and the oblique long process below (4) are reliable landmarks in the diagnosis of ear disease. The light reflection ('light reflex') (5) is seen in the anterior inferior quadrant.

The fibrous tympanic annulus (*arrows*) is seen clearly in the inferior, anterior and posterior quadrants but it is absent superiorly in the region of the pars flaccida. The blood supply of the tympanic membrane is from superiorly: the so-called vascular strip (6). The recesses for the round window (7) and eustachian tube (8) can be seen behind this translucent drumhead.

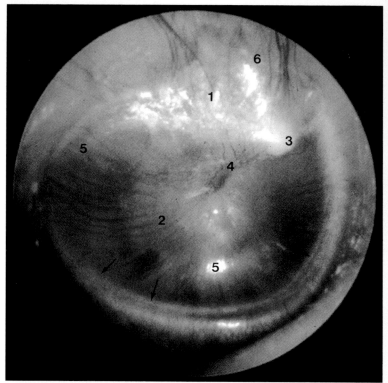

5 Normal middle ear An endoscopic view of a normal middle ear can be seen from the area of the orifice of the eustachian tube. A basic understanding of middle ear anatomy is necessary before one can interpret findings during otoscopy.

The tympanic membrane is conical, with its apex attached to the lower end of the malleus (1) at the umbo. A fibrous tympanic annulus (2) serves as the attachment point of the tympanic membrane; the annulus is very thin superiorly. The tensor tympani (3) inserts into the malleus behind the short process of the malleus (4). The chorda tympani (5) exits from the bone of the posterior wall of the middle ear and traverses through the tympanic cavity between the incus and malleus. The long process (6) of the incus ends in an enlarged process, the lenticular (7) or lens-shaped process. The lenticular process of the incus articulates with the capitulum (8) of the stapes. The stapedial tendon (9) inserts into the neck of the stapes. The facial nerve (10) can be seen immediately above and behind the stapes.

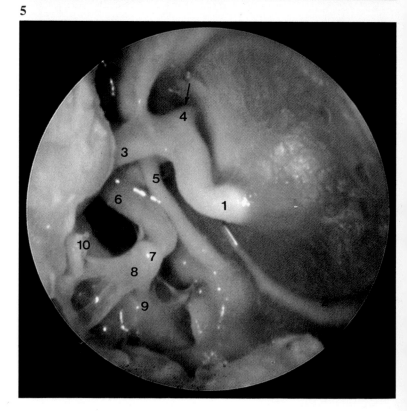

6 Normal left tympanic membrane The translucent character of the normal tympanic membrane can be seen even though some keratinization is visible on the surface of the drumhead in this case. Note the normal obliquity of the long process of the malleus. The umbo is the central attachment of the tympanic membrane to the malleus (*arrowed*).

6

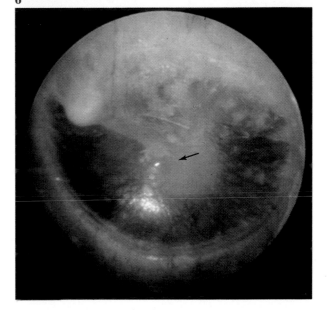

7 Normal right tympanic membrane The translucency of this tympanic membrane allows visualization of the underlying incus (1), eustachian tube orifice (2) and the round window niche (3). The anterior part of the tympanic annulus, the anterior sulcus (4), is often hidden from view during routine otoscopy.

7

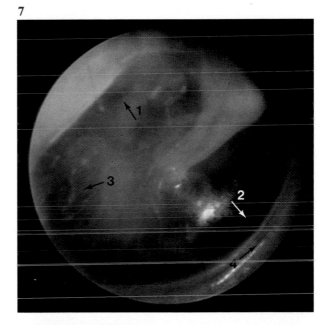

8 A tympanic membrane seen during conventional otoscopy for comparison purposes. The central portion of the tympanic membrane can be seen, including the long process of the malleus, the umbo and the long process of the incus (*left*). The majority of the tympanic membrane is not seen since the isthmus of the ear canal is appreciably smaller than the drumhead.

8

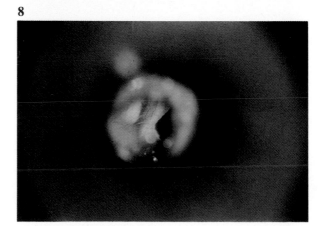

9

10

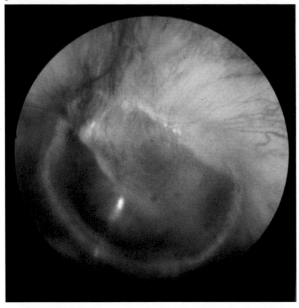

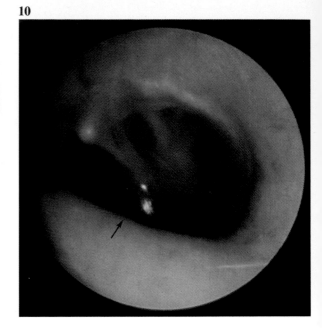

11

9   Normal left tympanic membrane In this normal tympanic membrane the major blood supply is visible coming from the ear canal superiorly – the 'vascular strip'. These blood vessels extend over the long process of the malleus and should not be confused with an inflammatory process.

10   Normal left tympanic membrane In this case a normal tympanic membrane is partly obscured by a prominent anterior external auditory canal wall (*arrowed*). In most cases, the anterior 1/3 of the tympanic membrane is obscured by the canal wall when viewed with conventional otoscopes.

11   Normal left tympanic membrane In this normal tympanic membrane, the incus is clearly visible behind the translucent membrane. The anterior sulcus is obscured by the prominent anterior canal wall.

12

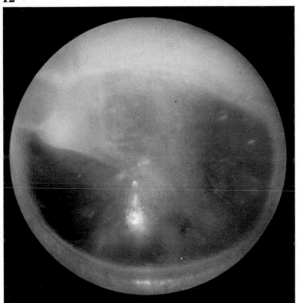

13

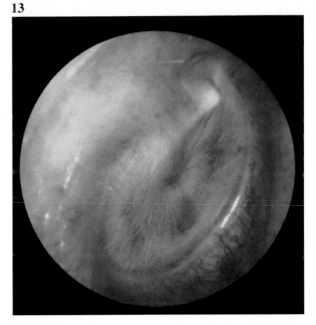

14

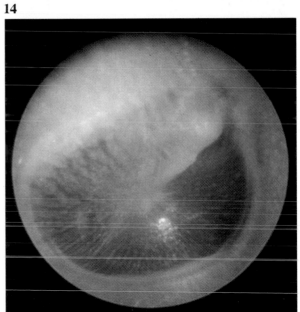

12   Normal left tympanic membrane This is the normal tympanic membrane of an 18-month-old child. Note the increased obliquity of the long process of the malleus which is often seen in young children.

13   Normal right tympanic membrane This normal tympanic membrane appears thicker than usual and the malleus is more vertical. Although this patient had no hearing loss or otologic disease, light reflection is not seen since no portion of the drumhead is perpendicular to the path of light from the otoscope.

14   Normal right tympanic membrane The translucency of this tympanic membrane is somewhat obscured by the keratinization of the surface epithelium – a normal variant.

External auditory canal

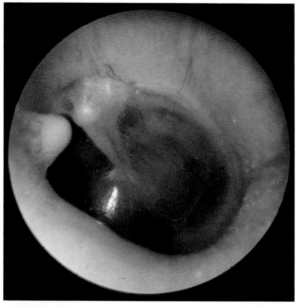

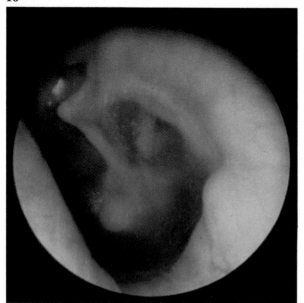

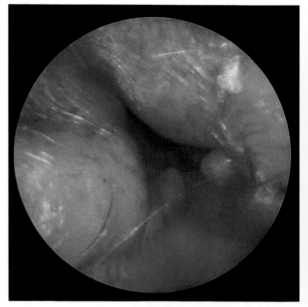

15 **Exostosis external auditory canal** A solitary exostosis is seen in the superior portion of the bony canal wall. This common finding is asymptomatic and not associated with hearing loss. It is hard when palpated with an instrument.

16 **Exostoses of external auditory canal** Multiple small exostoses are seen in the canal of this cold water swimmer. One exostosis appears to be arising from the promontory (medial wall of the middle ear) and touching the medial surface of the tympanic membrane.

17 **Multiple exostoses external auditory canal** This external canal is almost occluded by multiple sessile exostoses of the bony canal. Exostoses of this type are often seen in cold water swimmers. Some patients with multiple exostoses experience recurrent external otitis; in such cases surgical removal of the lesions is indicated.

18

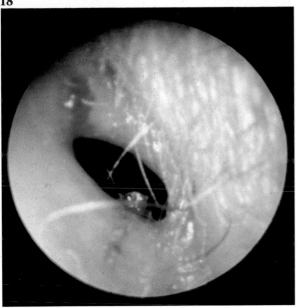

19

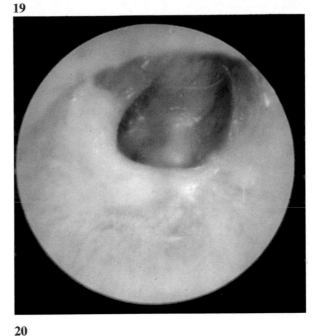

20

18 External auditory canal stenosis Stenosis of the external auditory canal may be congenital or acquired. This congenitally stenotic canal was 1mm x 2mm in size and associated with ossicular fixation. Canal stenosis may follow recurrent external otitis or trauma.

19 External auditory canal stenosis A temporal bone fracture extending to the external auditory canal resulted in a web-like stenosis in this ear, with a lumen size of 1.5mm.

20 External canal seborrheic dermatitis This patient has longstanding seborrhea with recurrent pruritis of the external canal. The canal wall is dry, scaly and excoriated. These patients are effectively treated with topical corticosteroids.

21

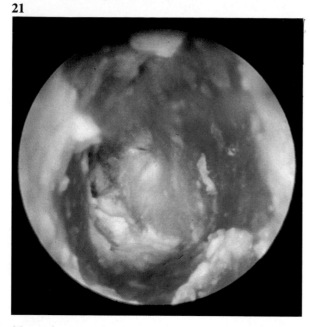

22

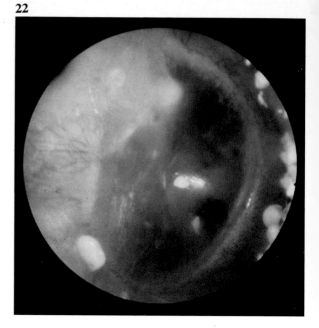

23

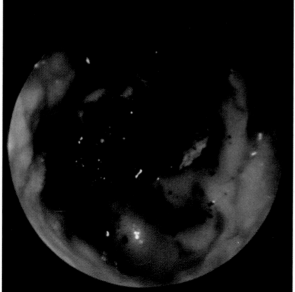

21 Acute external otitis Acute bacterial external otitis is a common disorder usually caused by *Staphylococcus aureus* or *Pseudomonas aeruginosa*. In this case a copious, creamy exudate fills the medial canal. The underlying skin is erythematous and oedematous.

22 Saprophytic fungi of the external canal Small yellow-white colonies of fungi are seen in this child's external canal. This incidental finding requires no therapy.

23 Otomycosis Exudate and black mycelia are seen in this case of external otitis due to *Aspergillis niger*.

24

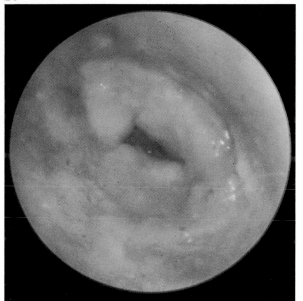

25

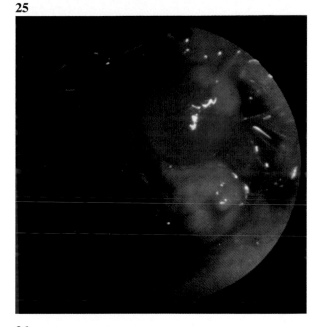

26

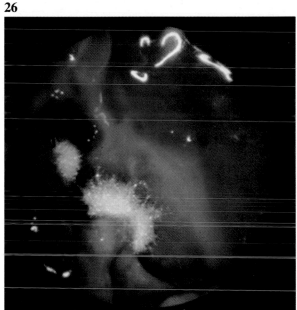

24 Acute external otitis In this case of acute bacterial external otitis, purulent debris totally occludes the external canal. The yellow-green to blue-green colour and characteristic odour lead one to suspect *Pseudomonas*, which was confirmed on culture.

25 Necrotizing external otitis Necrotizing external otitis (malignant external otitis) is a rare infection of the temporal bone due to *Pseudomonas aeruginosa*. It is seen typically in elderly diabetics and is characterised by granulation tissue and necrosis in the external auditory canal. Early recognition and aggressive medical and surgical therapy may cure this potentially lethal disease.

26 Infected mastoid cavity After radical mastoid surgery a large cavity may fill with epithelial debris which may become infected. In this case, purulent debris and granulation tissue are present in a large mastoid 'bowl'. Fungal growth, seen here as a white and cotton-like material, is a frequent secondary infection.

27

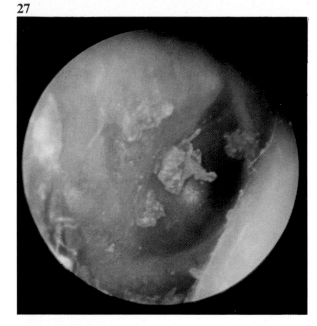

28

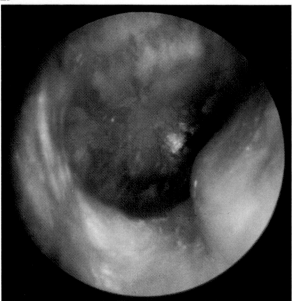

29

27 Debris on the tympanic membrane Although cerumen is produced only in the lateral one-third of the external auditory canal it is often found on the drumhead due to manipulation with hairpins or cotton tipped applicators, as in this case.

28 Keratosis obturans An abnormal, accelerated buildup of keratin (*arrows*) has led to bone erosion in the floor of the external auditory canal. This uncommon disease has been observed in association with bronchiectasis and sinusitis, but its aetiology is unknown.

29 Keratosis obturans Longstanding keratosis obturans has led to extensive bone loss on the floor of the external canal. The keratin had been removed preceding the photograph.

30

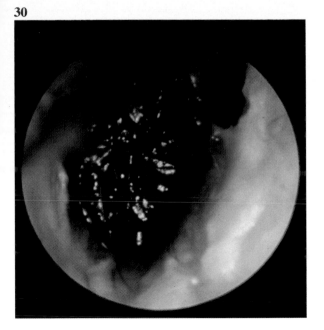

31

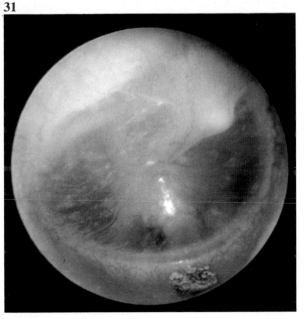

32

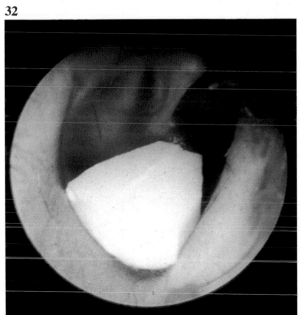

30   Cerumen impaction An abnormal accumulation of cerumen has occluded this external auditory canal. Cerumen impactions are often the result of manipulation of the external canal with cotton-tipped applicators or hair pins. Such manipulation forces cerumen medial to the narrow isthmus of the ear canal, where it cannot be cleared by the normal lateral flow of cerumen.

31   Foreign body – external auditory canal A small sand particle can be seen just below the tympanic annulus. Foreign bodies of this type are common in children and are usually cleared from the ear canal by normal lateral epithelial migration from the tympanic membrane.

32   Foreign body – external auditory canal A fragment of a bean from a beanbag was lodged in this child's ear. Instrumentation of such foreign bodies may injure the tympanic membrane or lacerate the ear canal. These foreign bodies must be removed with adequate light and illumination, sometimes with general anaesthesia. Specially adapted suction apparatus is a particularly atraumatic means of removing foreign bodies of the ear canal.

Myringitis

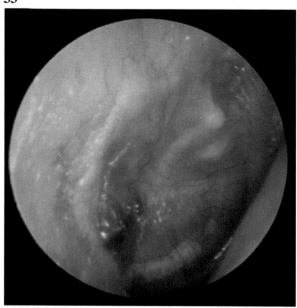

33 Acute bullous myringitis (early) This patient complained of an acute onset of severe right ear pain without fever or chills. Small vesicles are seen on the inferior portion of the tympanic membrane. The drumhead is mobile.

34 Acute bullous myringitis (late) Bullous myringitis is an acute, painful, inflammatory disease of the tympanic membrane. Multiple bullae are seen on the drum surface, which may contain blood or exudate. This condition is thought to be of viral origin, but *Mycoplasma pneumoniae* has been cultured. Bullae may be seen in early acute otitis media.

35 Herpes zoster oticus Herpes Zoster Oticus (Ramsey Hunt Syndrome) is an Herpes zoster infection of the seventh cranial nerve. In this case, vesicles are seen involving the medial ear canal and tympanic membrane. Peripheral facial nerve paralysis is seen in many cases.

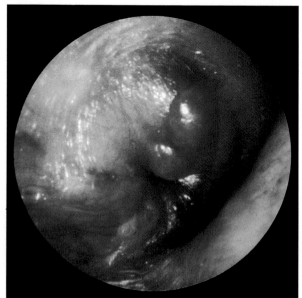

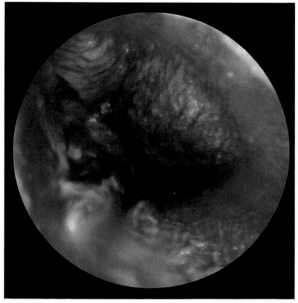

36

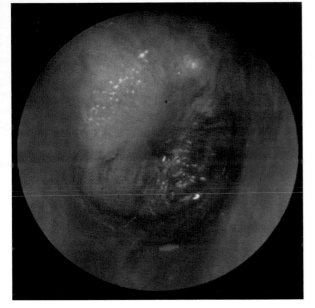

37

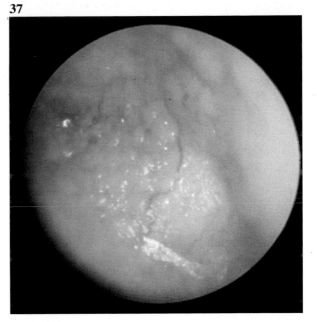

38

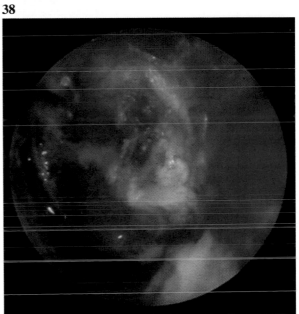

36   Granular myringitis A diffuse, granular, irregular appearance is seen in this patient, who had been using otic drops excessively. This inflammatory reaction is due to a sensitivity to Neomycin.

37   Granular myringitis A diffuse granularity of a grafted tympanic membrane is seen on another patient who uses otic drops excessively.

38   Granular myringitis A longstanding external otitis has resulted in an accumulation of granulation tissue in the tympanic membrane and the medial portion of the external canal.

Acute otitis media

39 Normal tympanic membrane – prior to otitis media Figures 39 through 47 are photographs of the right tympanic membrane of a 2½-year-old child who experienced a bout of acute otitis media with resolution. Prior to the infection the tympanic membrane appeared normal, although this patient had occasional bouts of serous otitis media.

40 Early acute purulent otitis media (*see* **39-47**) Shortly after the onset of right otalgia the tympanic membrane appeared erythematous and slightly bulging. Yellow purulent material was seen behind the drumhead. It was treated with oral Ampicillin. The most frequent causative organisms in acute otitis media are *Streptococcus pneumoniae*, *Streptococcus viridans* and *Haemophilis influenzae*. *H. influenzae* is a significant pathogen only in children.

41 Acute purulent otitis media (*see* **39-47**) Twelve hours after the onset of acute otitis media the drumhead is bulging and the middle ear is filled with purulent material. The light reflex is seen easily in this case of acute otitis and is therefore not a reliable sign in otologic diagnosis.

39

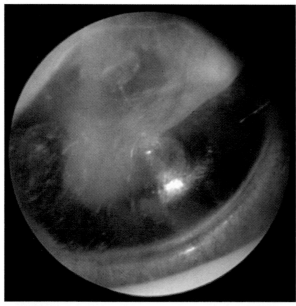

40

41

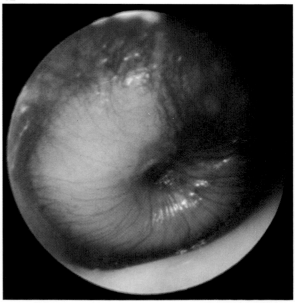

42

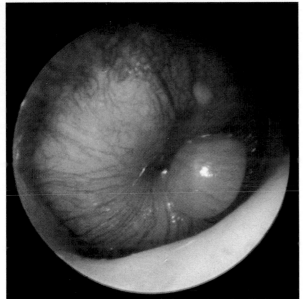

43

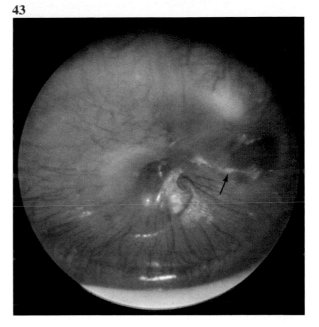

44

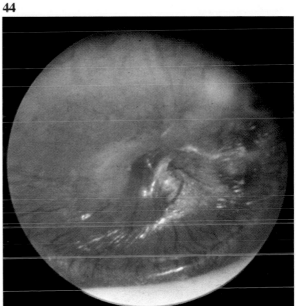

42   Acute purulent otitis media – day 2 (*see* **39-47**)
Two days after the onset of acute otitis media a bleb
appeared in the antero-inferior portion of the tympanic
membrane: an impending perforation. At this stage
acute otitis media may be confused with bullous
myringitis.

43 Acute purulent otitis media – day 3 (*see* **39-47**)
Three days after the onset of acute otitis media the
previously seen bleb had ruptured and a crust formed in
that area. An air bubble (*arrowed*) is now visible behind
the anterior portion of the tympanic membrane.

44   Acute purulent otitis media – day 6 (*see* **39-47**)
Six days after the onset of acute otitis media more air
bubbles are visible behind the drumhead as the purulent
material is absorbed.

45

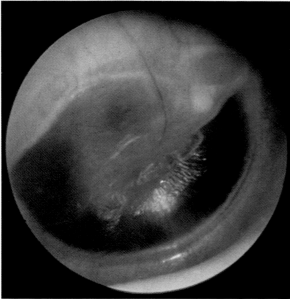

46

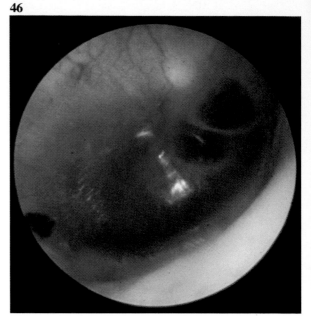

47

45 Acute purulent otitis media – day 10 (*see* **39-47**) Ten days after the onset of acute otitis media the middle ear is air containing and a yellowish crust is visible over the area which had been perforated previously.

46 Acute purulent otitis media – day 20 (*see* **39-47**) After resolution of acute otitis media, a middle ear effusion may persist for weeks to months. In this case a serous middle ear effusion persisted for one month.

47 Acute purulent otitis media – resolved (*see* **39-47**) After six months the episode of acute otitis media has resolved and the tympanic membrane is normal.

48
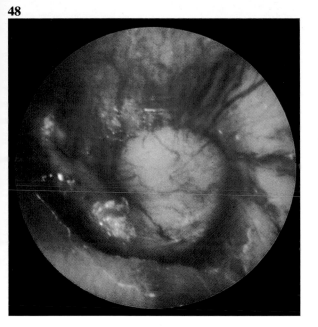

49
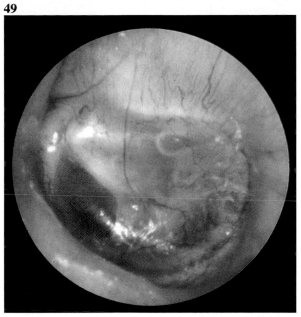

50
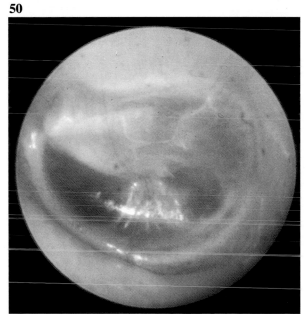

48 Acute purulent otitis media Acute otitis media in the left ear of an adult. Erythema of the drumhead and surrounding canal with a bulging tympanic membrane are the hallmarks of this disease.

49 Acute purulent otitis media – one week After one week of antibiotics, the purulent middle ear effusion has become serous and an air bubble is visible posterior to the malleus.

50 Acute purulent otitis media – resolved Two weeks after a course of antibiotics the middle ear effusion has cleared and the tympanic membrane appears normal. The angulation of the long process of the malleus is unusual but not abnormal.

51   Acute purulent otitis media Acute otitis media of the right tympanic membrane. The middle ear is filled with purulent material and the drumhead is bulging. Erythema is most marked over the malleus and superior ear canal.

51

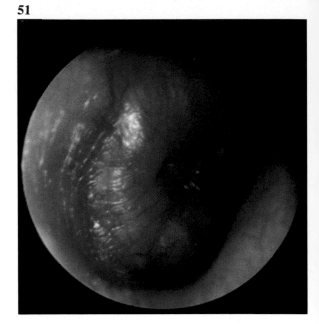

52   Acute purulent otitis media An horizontal section of a temporal bone showing acute otitis media. A purulent effusion surrounds the incus (1). Mucosal thickening and fibrosis (2) is also present.

52

53   Acute purulent otitis media In this temporal bone section, acute otitis media has led to extreme mucosal thickening over the cochlea (1) and also surrounds the incus (2) and malleus (3).

53

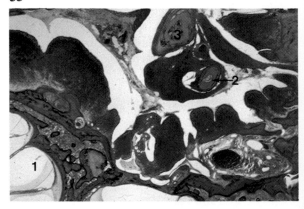

Tympanosclerosis

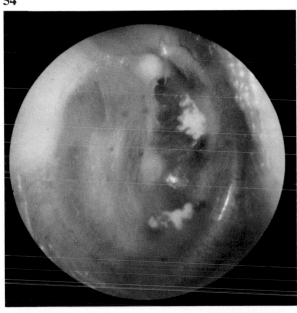

54 **Mild tympanosclerosis** Tympanosclerosis is a common sequel of acute otitis media. It is recognised by chalky, white deposits in the tympanic membrane. Two small patches of tympanosclerosis are seen in the anterior quadrants of this right tympanic membrane. Contrastingly, there is scarring and collagen formation in the posterior quadrants.

55 **Mild tympanosclerosis** Patches of mild tympanosclerosis are evident in the posterior quadrants; there was no associated hearing loss.

56 **Tympanosclerosis** The typical crescentic pattern of tympanosclerosis is seen in this left tympanic membrane. In most cases tympanosclerosis is limited to the tympanic membrane and does not affect hearing.

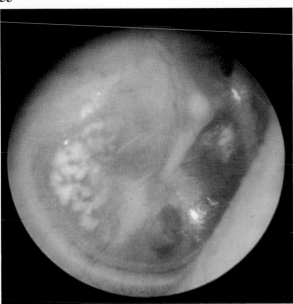

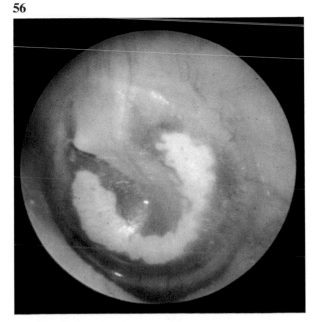

57

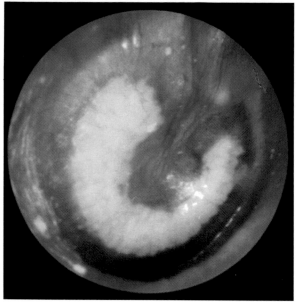

57 Tympanosclerosis Another example of the chalky plaques of tympanosclerosis. This patient has been observed for fifteen years with no change in the plaques or deterioration of hearing.

58

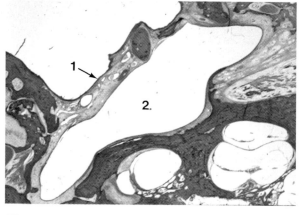

58 Tympanosclerosis – histopathology Longstanding tympanosclerosis involving the tympanic membrane (1) and middle ear (2). Note the eosinophilic, hyaline deposits in the middle layer of the tympanic membrane and also submucosally over the cochlea.

59

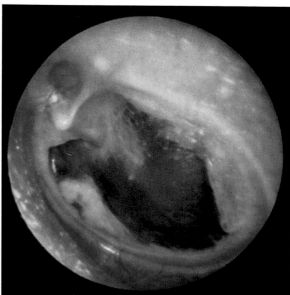

59 Tympanosclerosis In this case mild tympanosclerosis was seen on otoscopy which was associated with a conductive hearing loss. Extensive tympanosclerosis was found to fix the stapes at surgery. Tympanosclerosis involving the ossicles may or may not be heralded by plaques on the tympanic membrane.

60

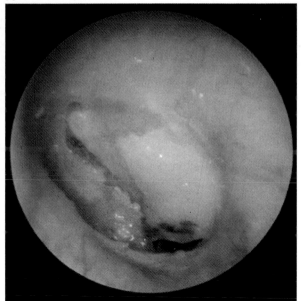

61

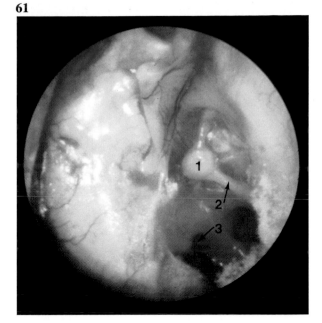

62

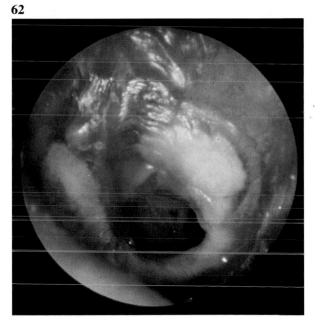

60 Severe tympanosclerosis Tympanosclerosis involves the entire tympanic membrane in this patient with an 18 dB conductive hearing loss. A small perforation can be seen at the inferior portion of this tympanic membrane.

61 Severe tympanosclerosis Severe tympanosclerosis can be seen in the anterior half of the left tympanic membrane. Posteriorly, the tympanic membrane is very thin and adherent to the capitulum of the stapes (1) – spontaneous myringostapediopexy; the incus has been eroded. The stapedius tendon (2) and the round window (3) are also visible through the thin membrane.

62 Tympanosclerosis with perforation In this left tympanic membrane, prior inflammation has left a moderate size perforation and thick tympanosclerosis in the remaining tympanic membrane.

63 Tympanosclerosis with perforations As a sequel of repeated otitis media this tympanic membrane has two perforations (*arrowed*), extensive white tympanosclerosis and an attachment of the remaining drumhead to the incus – spontaneous myringoincudopexy (1).

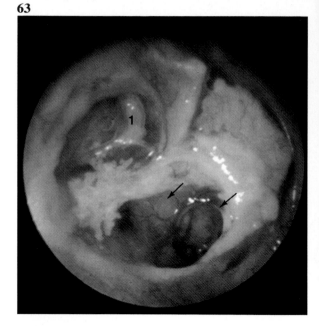

64 Obliterative tympanosclerosis This ear is extensively affected by tympanosclerosis of the tympanic membrane and middle ear. Middle ear tympanosclerosis is visible through a large perforation in this left tympanic membrane. This patient had a 55 dB conductive hearing loss due to obliteration of the oval window with tympanosclerotic plaques.

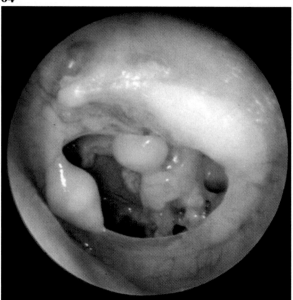

65 Obliterative tympanosclerosis–histopathology Tympanosclerosis and new bone formation fills the middle ear and surrounds the stapes (*arrow*).

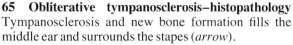

Traumatic perforation

66 Traumatic perforation – day one (*see* **66-68**) These left tympanic membrane perforations were caused by an accidental blow to the side of the head. One small perforation is seen just below the umbo and posterior to the light reflection. Another large perforation in the posterior part of the tympanic membrane exposes the round window niche.

67 Traumatic perforation – day 14 (*see* **66-68**) The injured tympanic membrane shown in **66** was allowed to heal spontaneously. After fourteen days the small perforation below the umbo has healed and the large posterior perforation is smaller. Infolding of the margins of traumatic perforations may rarely lead to cholesteatoma formation.

68 Traumatic perforation – day 42 (*see* **66-68**) The traumatised left tympanic membrane shown in **66** and **67** has completely healed without treatment in six weeks. Most traumatic perforations heal spontaneously without surgical intervention.

66

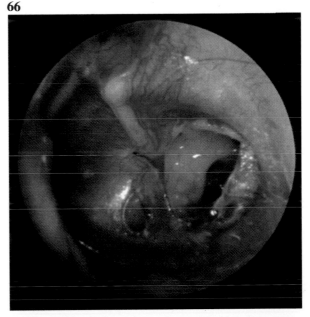

67

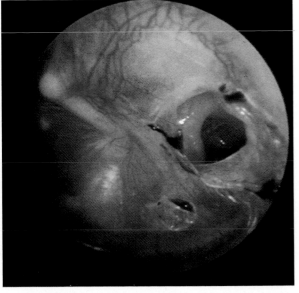

68

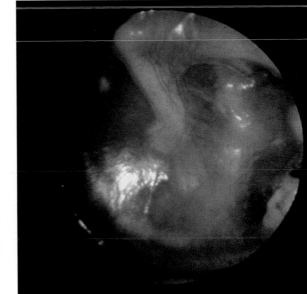

69

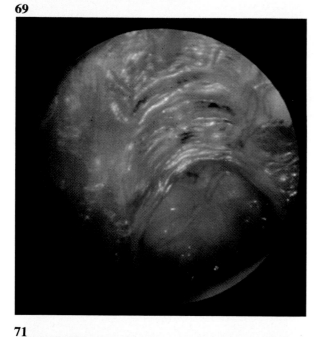

70

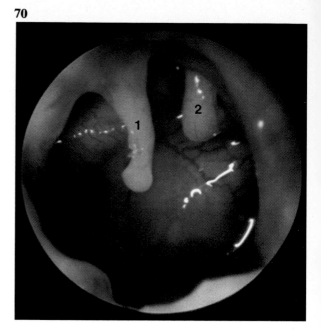

71

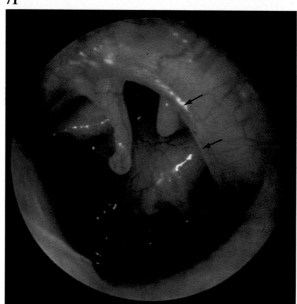

69 Traumatic perforation This right tympanic membrane perforation was a result of a blow to the side of the head in a young man. In contradistinction to the case shown in **66-68**, this tympanic membrane has not healed after six months. The tympanic annulus is deficient antero-inferiorly and the perforation is large; these two factors make spontaneous healing unlikely.

70 Traumatic perforation – total (*see* **70 & 71**) The entire tympanic membrane was lost after hot grease was poured into this man's left ear. The long process of the malleus (1) and the incus (2) is clearly visible. The middle ear mucosa is inflamed and oedematous.

71 Traumatic perforation – total (*see* **70 & 71**) After four months the perforation shown in **70** has shown little sign of healing. The middle ear mucosa is more normal in appearance and there is a minimal attempt at healing near the posterior-superior tympanic annulus (*arrows*).

72 **73**

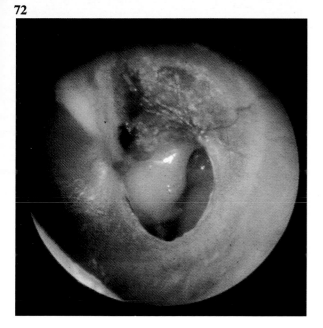

72   Traumatic perforation Two days after a blow to the left side of the head, this patient was found to have a moderate sized tympanic membrane perforation. A 23 dB conductive hearing loss was documented audiometrically. This perforation healed without therapy.

73   Traumatic perforation – iatrogenic This patient underwent a successful stapedectomy ten years previously but a perforation was seen in the postoperative period. Evidently the tympanic annulus (*arrow*) was pulled anteriorly and a small perforation developed between the fibrous and bony annulus.

Chronic perforations

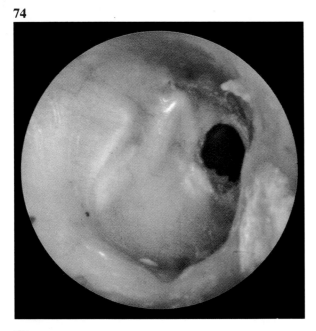

74

74 Perforation This is an asymptomatic simple perforation of the right tympanic membrane anterior to the long process of the malleus. This tympanic membrane is thickened due to repeated infections many years previously; hearing was normal.

75 Subtotal perforation A large perforation of the left tympanic membrane due to repeated otitis media. The perforation exposes the round window niche, the long process of the incus and the tympanic orifice of the eustachian tube.

76 Perforation Small perforations of this type can become repeatedly infected. In this case a small area of granulation tissue can be seen on the posterior margin of the left tympanic membrane perforation. The thickening and tympanosclerosis of the remainder of the drumhead are a sequela of prior infection.

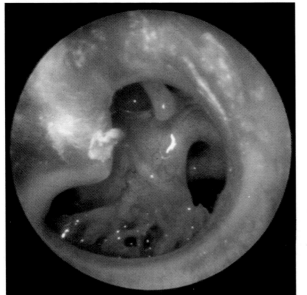

75

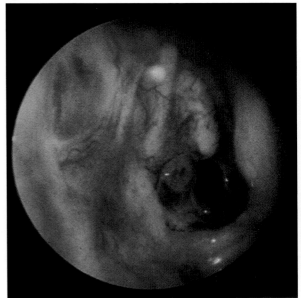

76

77

78

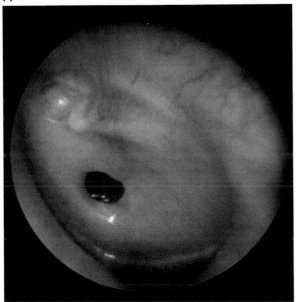

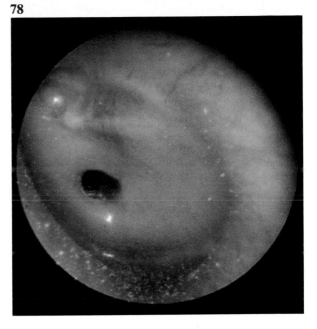

77 Possible perforation (*see* **78**) At first examination, it was thought that there was a small perforation in the anterior portion of this thickened right tympanic membrane. This patient was asymptomatic and had no hearing loss.

78 Neomembrane simulating a perforation (*see* **77**) After the drumhead shown in **77** was powdered, a few particles of powder adhered to the neomembrane. Perforations of the tympanic membrane often heal with a very thin neomembrane. These thin, clear areas are frequently confused with perforations; such an area may be distinguished with the pneumatic otoscope or under the microscope.

79

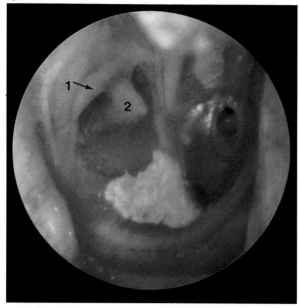

80

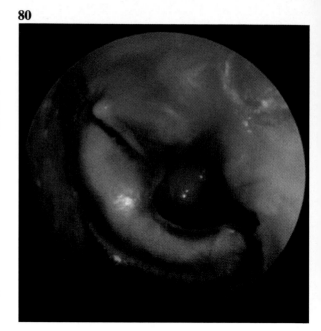

81

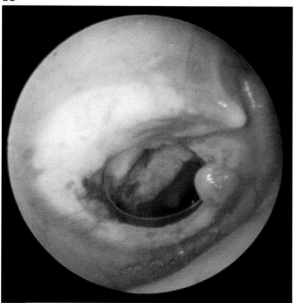

79 Perforation and tympanosclerosis A small perforation resulted from an episode of right acute otitis media. This perforation is out of the view of conventional otoscopes because of a prominent anterior canal wall. A large plaque of tympanosclerosis is present just below the umbo. The chorda tympani (1) is clearly visible coursing over the incus (2) and behind the malleus.

80 Perforation and tympanosclerosis A moderate size perforation is seen in this left tympanic membrane which is heavily infiltrated with tympanosclerosis. The round window niche is visible through the tympanic membrane. Exposure of the round window is associated with a conductive hearing loss since the pressure equalizing function of the round window is voided by the action of sound waves upon the window.

81 Perforation and tympanosclerosis In this case, tympanosclerosis and perforation were the result of repeated otitis media over many years. Tympanosclerotic plaques are seen in the drumhead as well as the middle ear.

82

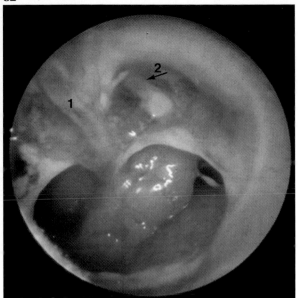

83

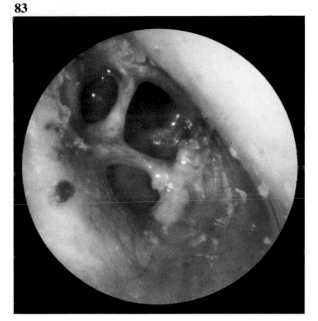

84

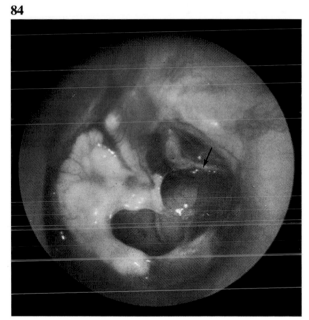

82 Perforation This large inferior perforation is the result of chronic otitis media. The malleus (1) is retracted and adherent to the promontory. Adhesions between the malleus and the promontory are a common cause of conductive hearing loss due to otitis media. The retracted posterior-superior portion of this drumhead is adherent to the long process of the incus (2) forming a spontaneous myringoincudopexy.

83 Multiple perforations Multiple perforations of a right tympanic membrane due to recurrent otitis media are evident here. Multiple perforations have been associated with tuberculous otitis in the past, but recent reports describe large perforations with purulent drainage.

84 Multiple perforations Recurrent otitis media has led to two perforations, tympanosclerosis and a spontaneous myringoincudopexy in this right ear. The stapedius tendon (*arrowed*) can be seen extending from the capitulum of the stapes, below the incus, to the pyramidalis process to the right.

85

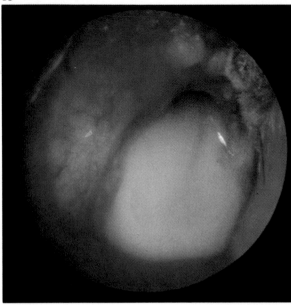

86

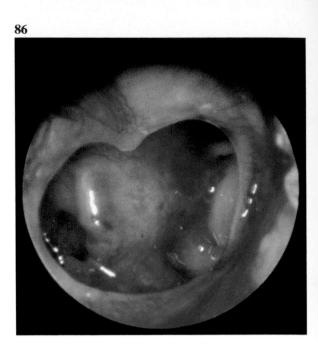

87

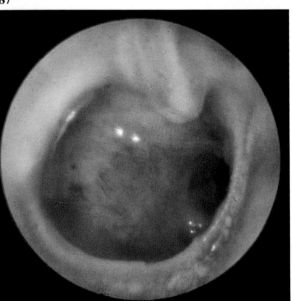

85   Infected perforation Grossly purulent material is seen in this large right tympanic membrane perforation. The unsuspecting examiner might assume that such a case represents an external otitis. Careful examination and follow-up are necessary in order to avoid overlooking a perforation in such a case.

86   Infected perforation Purulent material is seen in the middle ear of this patient with chronic otitis and otorrhea. The most common organisms cultured in this type of ear are *Pseudomonas* and *Staphylococcus*.

87   Infected perforation This near total perforation was the result of a necrotising otitis media. In this photograph, the middle ear is filled with purulent material; *Pseudomonas aeruginosa* was cultured.

88

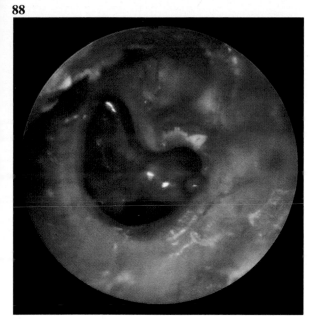

89

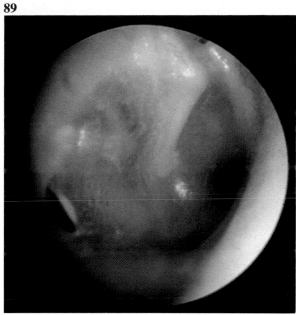

90

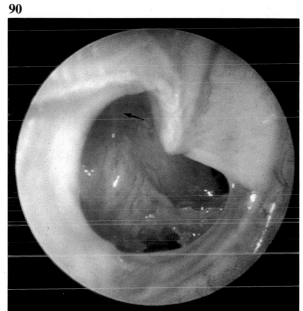

88 Perforation This longstanding perforation produces an almost constant mucoid otorrhea. Mucous glands in the middle ear of chronically infected ears may lead to otorrhea even in the absence of culturable organisms.

89 Perforation A small perforation of the right tympanic membrane of a child in whom a myringotomy grommet had been removed. Epithelial healing of the margins of this perforation has prevented spontaneous closure.

90 Perforation A dry, subtotal perforation of the right tympanic membrane. The long process of the incus and the suprastructure of the stapes are absent (*arrowed*).

91

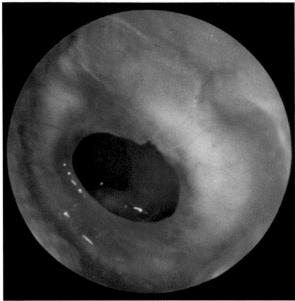

92

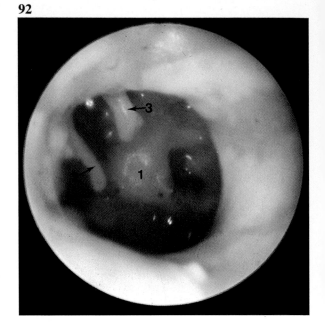

93

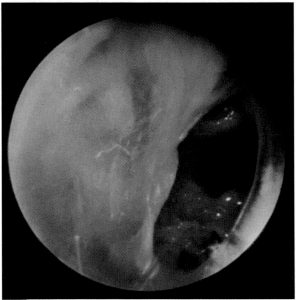

91 Chronic perforation This chronic perforation of a left tympanic membrane is due to an episode of acute otitis media ten years previously. During the preceding year this ear had become infected repeatedly. The middle ear mucosa is oedematous and inflamed.

92 Chronic perforation A total perforation of the right tympanic membrane resulted from acute necrotising otitis media. In this case the mucosa of the middle ear sloughed, leaving bare bone on the promontory of the middle ear (1). The long process of the incus (2) and malleus (3) are clearly seen.

93 Chronic perforation This marginal perforation of the anterior half of a right tympanic membrane has exposed the eustachian tube orifice. Perforations involving the tympanic annulus are considered as unsafe since the keratinising epithelium of the drumhead and ear canal may grow down into the middle ear and thus lead to cholesteatoma.

94

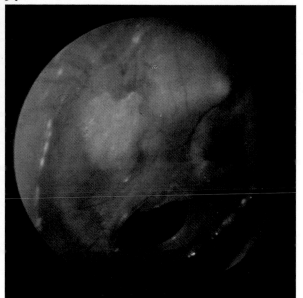

95

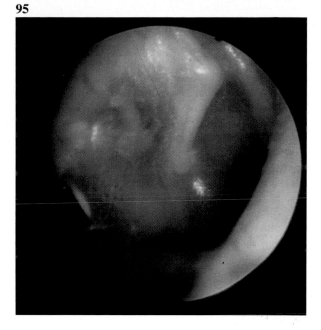

94 Chronic perforation This small perforation of a right tympanic membrane was the result of otitis media. The epithelium of the margin of the perforation has healed and the perforation has not closed. Most perforations of this size heal without therapy.

95 Persistent perforation This small posterior perforation persisted after removal of a myringotomy tube. Rapid epithelialisation of the margins of the perforation and persistent eustachian tube dysfunction may lead to persistent small perforations of this type.

Serous otitis media

96 Serous otitis media with effusion (OME) Serous otitis media (otitis media with effusion) is often seen as a sequelae of acute otitis media. Bacteria may be cultured in 25 to 30% of serous or mucinous middle ear effusions. Serous otitis media also occurs commonly without a history of otitis media; mechanical obstruction of the eustachian tube will lead to a middle ear effusion. In this case of a chronic effusion in a nine-year-old child, an amber coloured fluid is visualised behind a normal tympanic membrane. Gas bubbles are seen just anterior to the malleus. The light reflection (light reflex) is normal, as it is in most cases of otitis media with effusion.

97 Serous otitis media An histological preparation shows a child's temporal bone with serous otitis media. A serous effusion in the middle ear (*arrows*) is seen without inflammatory cells, although PMNs are sometimes seen in middle ear aspirates.

98 Serous otitis media A clear, amber coloured fluid is seen behind this right tympanic membrane. Several gas bubbles are visible, both anterior and posterior to the malleus. The erythema over the long process of the malleus should not be confused with the erythema associated with acute otitis media.

96

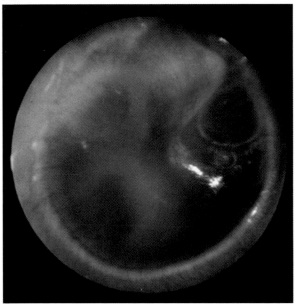

97

98

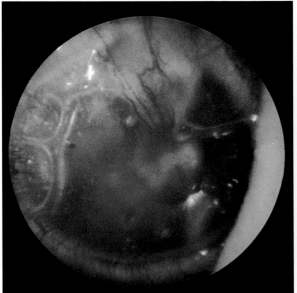

99

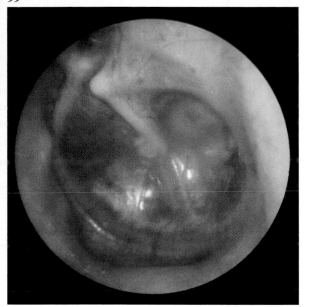

100

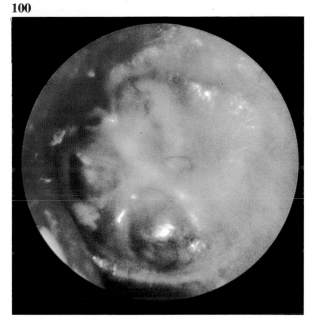

101

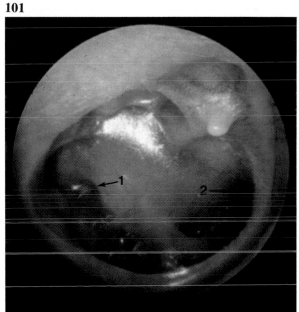

99 Serous otitis media This is an example of a longstanding left middle ear effusion in a six-year-old child. The entire pars tensa and pars flaccida are retracted medially and the middle ear cleft is filled with fluid; this child has a 25 dB conductive hearing loss. The paucity of abnormal findings on otoscopy is a feature of this disease; a middle ear effusion is suspected when the drumhead fails to move on pneumotoscopy.

100 Serous otitis media Repeated bouts of acute otitis media have resulted in a chronic middle ear effusion in this scarred left tympanic membrane. Retracted portions of the drumhead are most easily observed anterior to the malleus in this case.

101 Serous otitis media A lifelong history of middle ear effusion has resulted in a severely eroded malleus in this right ear of a 32-year-old woman. Not only is the long process of the malleus almost totally gone, but the remaining drumhead is retracted onto the medial wall of the middle ear. The recess for the round window (1) and the eustachian tube (2) are seen behind the thinned pars tensa.

102

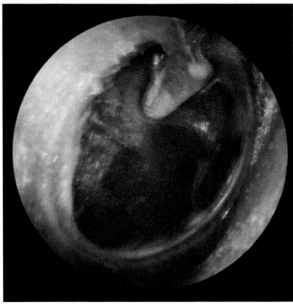

103

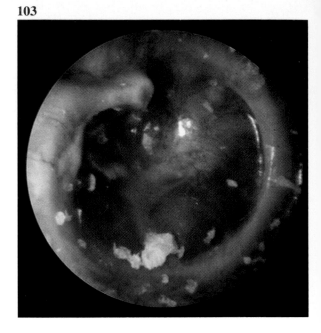

102 Mucoid otitis media (MOM) A chronic middle ear effusion in this right ear has led to erosion of the long process of the malleus. The thick mucoid fluid in the middle ear has led to a dark appearance of the drumhead. This type of an ear is sometimes called a 'glue ear' since the middle ear effusion resembles thick glue.

103 Mucoid otitis media Another longstanding middle ear effusion in this right ear has led to erosion of the entire long process of the malleus and severe retraction of the drumhead. The dark appearance of this type of chronic middle ear effusion has been mistakenly termed 'idiopathic haemotympanum' or 'blue eardrum'; there is no blood in this middle ear, rather, thick mucoid fluid.

104

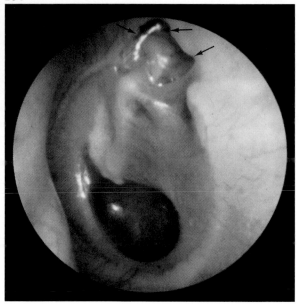

105

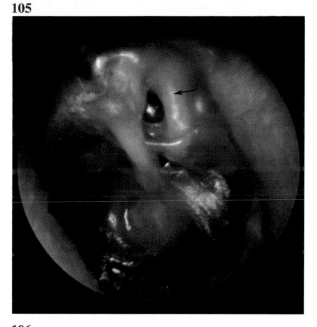

106

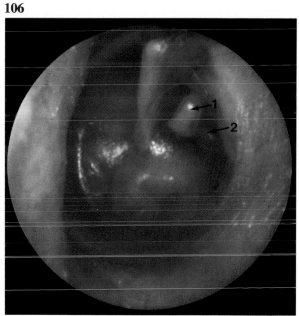

104 Serous otitis media with retraction A lifelong history of middle ear effusion in the left ear of this ten-year-old girl has led to progressive retraction of the pars tensa and pars flaccida. The retracted area is the area of the pars flaccida; bone erosion of the superior canal wall has occurred (*arrows*) and the head of the malleus is exposed. These retraction pockets may develop into cholesteatomas of the primary acquired type (*see* **119**).

105 Serous otitis media with retraction This severely retracted left tympanic membrane has almost totally collapsed the middle ear space. The long process of the incus (*arrow*) is covered by only a thin retracted membrane.

106 Serous otitis media with middle ear atelectasis Chronic serous otitis and recurrent acute otitis media has resulted in atelectasis of the middle ear. The thin drumhead is adherent to a partially eroded incus (1) (spontaneous myringoincudopexy) and the stapedial tendon is visible behind it (2).

107

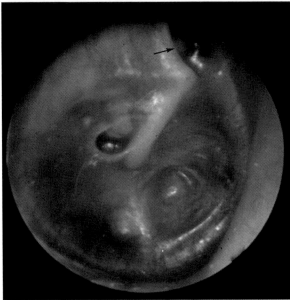

108

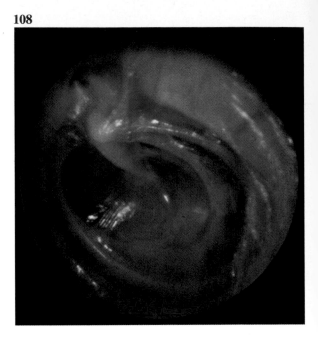

109

107 Serous otitis media Serous otitis media in the right ear of a three-year-old girl has been treated for two years. A prior myringotomy and intubation resulted in a thin, retracted area behind the long process of the malleus. Note the pars flaccida retraction pocket (*arrow*).

108 Serous otitis media This middle ear effusion has been present in a two-year-old child's left ear for four months following a bout of acute otitis media. Although the middle ear is filled with serous fluid, the light reflection appears normal.

109 Serous otitis media with ossicular erosion Erosion of the long process of the malleus and absence of the entire long process of the incus is due to chronic middle ear effusion in this child's right ear. The drumhead is adherent to the capitulum of the stapes (spontaneous myringostapediopexy).

110

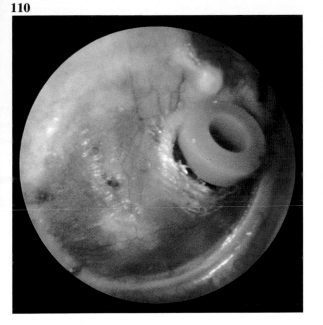

111

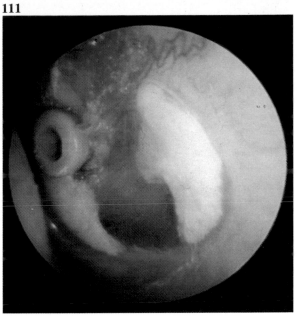

110 Myringotomy tube A myringotomy tube is seen just anterior to the malleus in this right tympanic membrane of a 2½-year-old boy with persistent serous otitis. These silicone tubes are retained in an opening in the drumhead by inner and outer flanges.

111 Myringotomy tube A myringotomy tube was placed in the anterior portion of this tympanic membrane. White tympanosclerotic plaques are the result of prior episodes of acute otitis media.

112

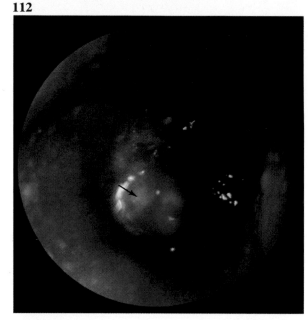

113

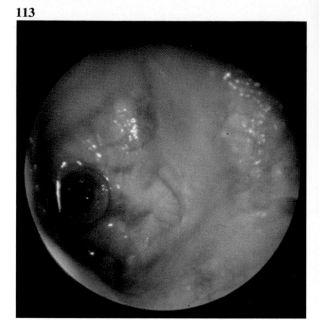

114

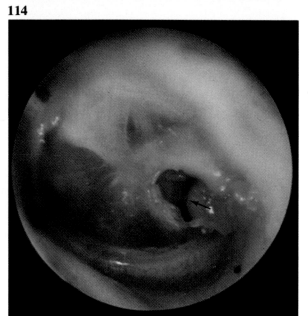

112 Myringotomy tube extrusion A previously placed myringotomy tube has extruded due to an episode of acute otitis media. Granulation tissue (*arrow*) is seen coming from the myringotomy, and the extruded silicone tube lies in the anterior sulcus.

113 Myringotomy tube with infection Purulent material is exuding from this myringotomy tube because of a bout of acute otitis media. Acute otitis in an intubated ear results in otorrhea with little pain or fever. Twenty percent of ears with tubes become acutely infected.

114 Myringotomy with cholesteatoma A myringotomy tube was extruded from this left tympanic membrane, resulting in a small perforation and a keratin pearl or cholesteatoma (*arrowed*). Cholesteatoma is a rare complication of myringotomy tubes.

Cholesteatoma

115

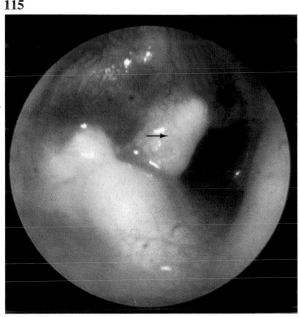

116

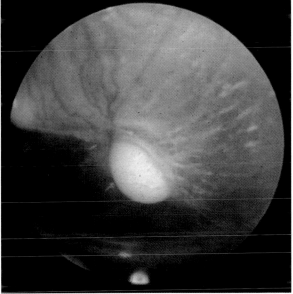

117

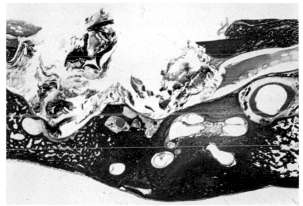

115 Congenital cholesteatoma A cholesteatoma of the middle ear or mastoid is an epidermal inclusion cyst lined with keratinising squamous epithelium. In this one-year-old child, a yellowish cholesteatoma was found in the lower one-half of the tympanic membrane. The upper part of the malleus (*arrow*) is visible in this right ear. Since there was no prior history of otitis, it is presumed that this is a rare congenital cholesteatoma due to a squamous epithelial rest in the middle ear.

116 Congenital cholesteatoma A small keratin pearl was found in the centre of this four-year-old's right tympanic membrane. There was no history of trauma or otitis media. These congenital keratin inclusion cysts may be the result of epithelial rests in the tympanic membrane.

117 Cholesteatoma An histological preparation of a temporal bone showing a large cholesteatoma: the darkly staining material is evident in the upper centre of the micrograph. As the cholesteatoma encounters bone, granulation tissue and bone erosion ensue. Cholesteatomas, regardless of origin, have a similar histopathological appearance.

118

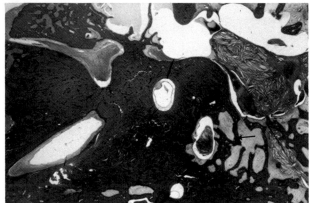

118 Cholesterol granuloma A cholesteatoma does not contain cholesterol; early investigators found the keratin grossly similar to cholesterol, hence the name. Cholesterol crystals are seen, however, in the middle ear and mastoid, even in the presence of cholesteatoma. This micrograph shows a cholesterol granuloma near mastoid air cells (*arrows*).

119

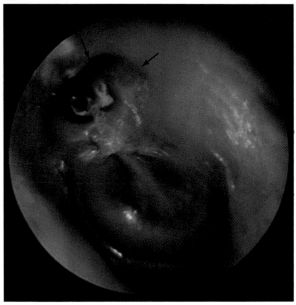

119 Primary acquired cholesteatoma A large cholesteatoma originated from this pars flaccida retraction pocket (*arrows*), and extended into the antrum and mastoid. A primary acquired cholesteatoma arises insidiously by gradual invagination of the pars flaccida. Some otologists believe that ingrowth of the basal layer of the epidermis of the pars flaccida causes these cholesteatomas. Although the exact pathogenesis of these common cholesteatomas is debated, they typically erode the posterior-superior canal wall and ossicles.

120

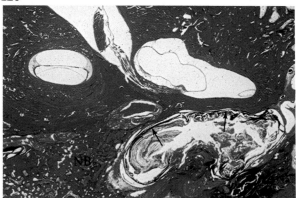

120 Cholesteatoma An histological preparation of another temporal bone with cholesteatoma shows areas of bone resorption (*arrows*) and areas of new bone formation (NB), probably related to recurrent infections.

121

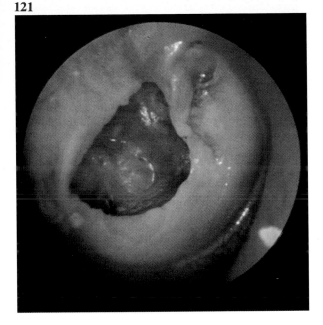

122

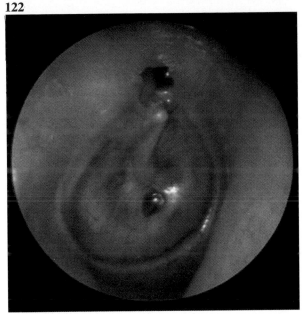

123

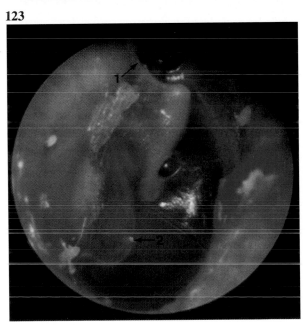

121 Primary acquired cholesteatoma A huge posterior retraction pocket is seen in this right ear. The incus and stapes have been eroded and a 40 dB conductive hearing loss is present. Although this 'retraction pocket' extends into the mastoid, as shown in mastoid X-rays, keratin has not been seen in this case over a four year period. Retraction pockets of this sort may erode bone, even in the absence of a keratin accumulation.

122 Pars flaccida retraction pocket A small retraction pocket is seen in this right ear in the area of the pars flaccida. Some otologists believe that this is the earliest stage in the development of primary acquired cholesteatoma. Bone erosion of the superior canal wall is minimal in this case. The retracted area below the umbo is the site of an healed perforation.

123 Primary acquired cholesteatoma A small cholesteatoma (1) is seen in this right ear. At the time of surgery, this cholesteatoma extended into the attic and antrum. This middle ear is filled with fluid and a gas bubble (2) can be seen behind the posterior part of the drumhead. Eustachian tube dysfunction is frequently seen in ears with cholesteatoma.

124

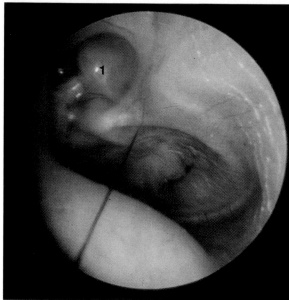

125

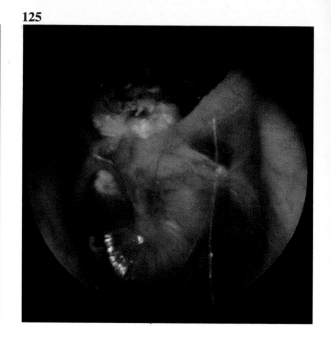

124 Primary acquired cholesteatoma Extensive bone erosion of the superior canal wall by this cholesteatoma has exposed the head of the malleus (1). At surgery this cholesteatoma extended to the antrum. Keratin filled the cholesteatoma, although it is not visible otoscopically.

125 Primary acquired cholesteatoma A large cholesteatoma is seen arising from the pars flaccida of this left tympanic membrane. The cholesteatoma has extensively eroded the superior canal wall and is filled with typical keratin debris.

126

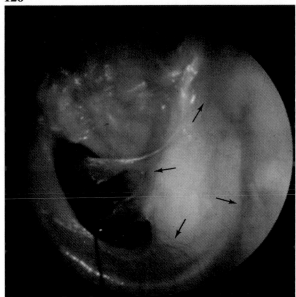

127

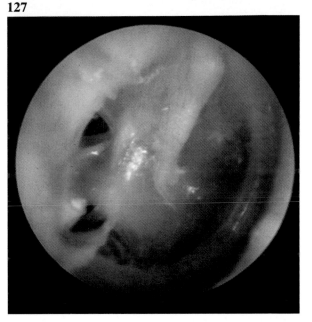

128

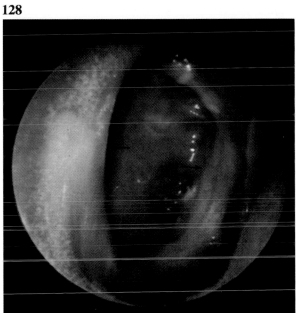

126 Cholesteatoma with perforation (Secondary acquired cholesteatoma) Secondary acquired cholesteatomas arise from the margins of large perforations due to otitis media. A large posterior perforation in the posterior half of this right tympanic membrane is associated with a rather large cholesteatoma in the anterior tympanic cavity (*arrows*). Cholesteatomas of this type are probably caused by an ingrowth of keratinising squamous epithelium from the margin of the perforation.

127 Cholesteatoma with perforation This small posterior perforation in a child's right ear was associated with a large cholesteatoma extending into the antrum and deep into the sinus tympani.

128 Potential cholesteatoma Keratinizing squamous epithelium has grown into the middle ear in this case of a right tympanic membrane perforation (*arrows*). This type of ingrowth of keratinising squamous epithelium into the middle ear depends upon damage to middle ear mucosa since at the contact point of these two types of epithelium, contact inhibition occurs and neither epithelium will overgrow the other.

129

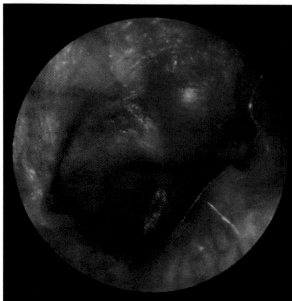

130

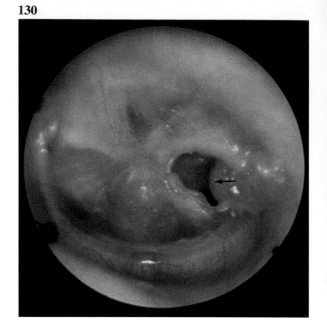

131

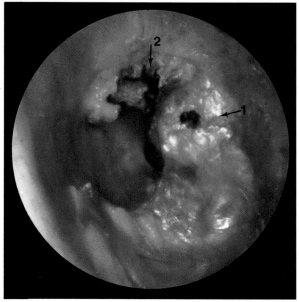

129 Cholesteatoma following trauma A cholesteatoma is seen in the posterior-superior portion of this right tympanic membrane. Three years previously, this patient sustained a traumatic perforation of this ear. Although the perforation healed spontaneously, a cholesteatoma developed behind this intact tympanic membrane, evidently as a result of implantation of keratinising squamous epithelium.

130 Cholesteatoma following myringotomy This small cholesteatoma (*arrow*) developed in this three-year-old child after the extrusion of a silicone ventilating tube. This cholesteatoma was most likely caused by an infolding of the surface squamous epithelium of the tympanic membrane. Cholesteatoma is a rare complication of middle ear ventilating tubes.

131 Cholesteatoma following surgery This right ear had a primary acquired cholesteatoma which was treated four years previously with an intact canal wall mastoidectomy and reconstruction with a polyethylene ossicular replacement prosthesis. The cholesteatoma has recurred and is seen as deeply retracted areas behind the prosthesis (1) and into the attic and antrum (2).

132

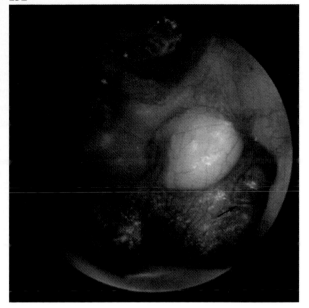

133

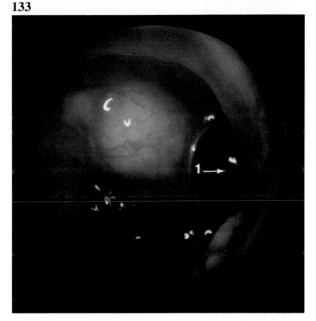

134

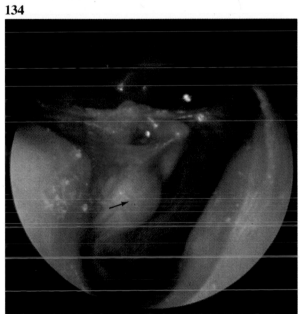

132 Recurrent cholesteatoma This cholesteatoma recurred in this child's left ear after radical mastoidectomy. The pearly cholesteatoma occurred in the areas of the oval window. A neomembrane has formed in the area of the eustachian tube orifice (*arrow*).

133 Recurrent cholesteatoma A cholesteatoma occurred in this six-year-old child's right ear one year after mastoidectomy. Persistent otorrhea was caused by infected, moist mucosa in the middle ear area. The eustachian tube orifice (1) and round window niche (2) are visible.

134 Recurrent cholesteatoma A cholesteatoma recurred in this right ear several years after modified radical mastoidectomy. The cholesteatoma (*arrows*) has occurred behind the long process of the malleus and was found enveloping the incus and stapes.

135

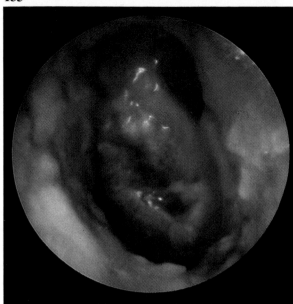

136

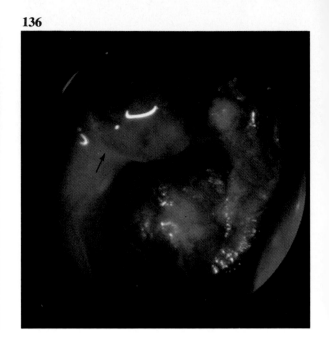

135 Infected cholesteatoma This infected cholesteatoma was mistakenly diagnosed as an external otitis. Careful examination, however, revealed an extensive area of superior canal erosion (*arrows*) filled with granulation tissue which heralds the cholesteatoma.

136 Infected cholesteatoma A polyp of granulation tissue (*arrows*) protrudes from the area of a cholesteatoma in this right ear. At the time of surgery a huge cholesteatoma was found extending into the antrum and mastoid air cells. Granulation tissue is frequently found in association with cholesteatoma. It is likely that this granulation tissue causes the bone erosion associated with cholesteatomas.

Postoperative findings

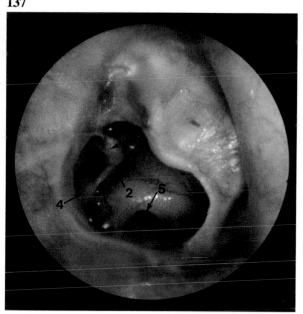

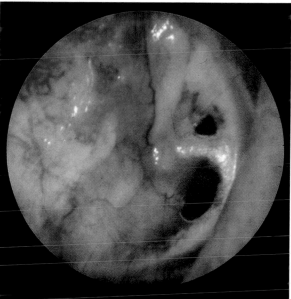

137 Tympanoplasty – prior to surgery (*see* **138**) A large right tympanic perforation exposes the incus (1), stapes (2), stapedial tendon (3), pyramidalis process (4), and round window niche (5). The anterior tympanosclerotic plaques involve the remaining drumhead. This patient had a conductive hearing loss with an air-bone gap of 25 dB.

138 Tympanoplasty – postoperative (*see* **137**) Six months after tympanoplasty the tympanic membrane is intact; the tympanosclerotic plaques were partially removed, leaving a thin anterior portion. The perforation was grafted with a temporalis fascia graft which appears as a thickened area to the left of the malleus. Postoperative hearing was improved; there was a 5 dB air-bone gap.

139

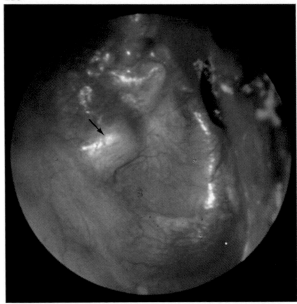

140

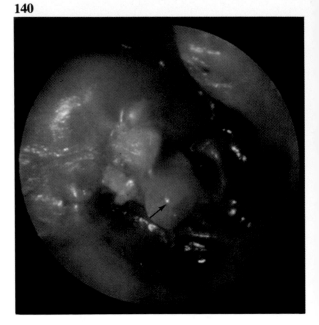

141

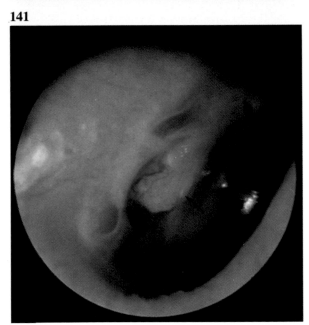

139 Tympanoplasty – incus transposition Three years after a right tympanoplasty, the grafted tympanic membrane appears thickened. The transposed incus (*arrow*) is visible beneath the graft. Postoperative hearing testing revealed a 22 dB air-bone gap.

140 Tympanoplasty – incus transposition This picture was taken two years after a right modified radical mastoidectomy and transposition of the incus (*arrow*) over the capitulum of the stapes. This patient has a 7 dB conductive hearing loss.

141 Tympanoplasty – incus transposition This patient underwent right ossicular reconstruction for erosion of the long process of the incus five years previously. The incus (*arrow*) was removed, then repositioned between the long process of the malleus and the stapes (*arrow*).

142

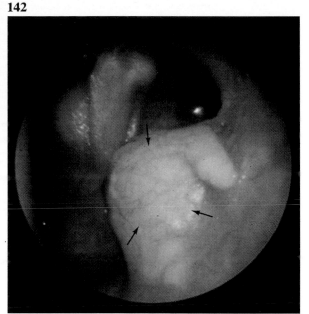

143

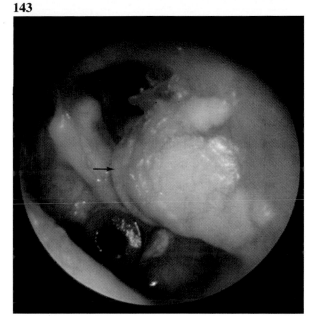

142 Tympanoplasty – polyethylene ossicular replacement strut (*see* **143**) This child had undergone a left intact canal wall mastoidectomy for cholesteatoma six months previously. Since the incus was involved in the cholesteatoma, it was removed and a texturised polyethylene strut was inserted between the stapes and the tympanic membrane; a piece of tragal cartilage (*arrows*) was placed over the plastic strut in an effort to prevent extrusion. At this point, recurrent eustachian tube dysfunction has led to retraction of the drumhead and middle ear effusion.

143 Tympanoplasty – polyethylene strut extrusion Three months after the photograph was taken and a myringotomy grommet was inserted, the polyethylene strut began to extrude (*arrowed*) and the cholesteatoma recurred.

144

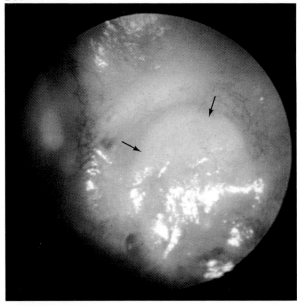

145

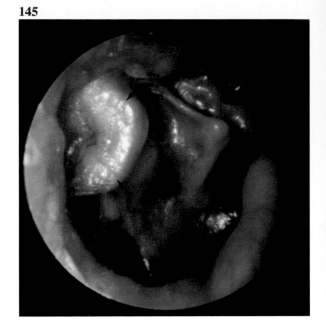

146

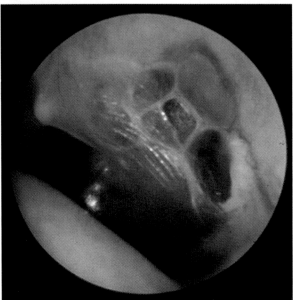

144 Tympanoplasty – cartilage strut This right ear had been reconstructed one year previously. The ossicular chain was reconstructed by using a self-stabilising cartilage strut. The round head of the cartilage strut is seen behind the drumhead (*arrows*).

145 Tympanoplasty – cartilage strut Because of the absence of the incus and the stapes, the sound conducting mechanism of this ear was reconstructed using a self-stabilising cartilage strut (*arrows*).

146 Postoperative stapedectomy Five years after a stapedectomy on this left ear, an area of scarring is visible in the posterior quadrants where the tympanic membrane was elevated during the surgical procedure. This scarring does not interfere with the sound conducting mechanism.

High jugular bulb

147   High jugular bulb (*see* **147-149**) The jugular
bulb is usually located just below the middle ear or the
labyrinth. In rare cases, such as those illustrated here,
the jugular bulb is exposed in the hypotympanic portion
of the middle ear and can be seen behind the inferior
portion of the tympanic membrane (*arrows*). This
thirteen-year-old girl complained of constant tinnitus in
her right ear. Surgical intervention, even simple
myringotomy, may result in serious haemorrhage in
these cases.

148   High jugular bulb (*see* **147 – 149**) This
computerised tomographic scan through the base of the
skull of the patient shown in figure 147 revealed a huge
jugular foramen on the right side (*arrows*) when com-
pared to the left side. The radiologist felt that this might
represent a glomus jugulare tumour, so a venogram was
performed to visualise the jugular vein.

149   High jugular bulb (*see* **147 – 149**) A right
jugular venogram was performed on the patient whose
ear is shown in figure **147**. A gross asymmetry was
found with a huge jugular vein and jugular bulb on the
right side. No therapy is indicated.

147

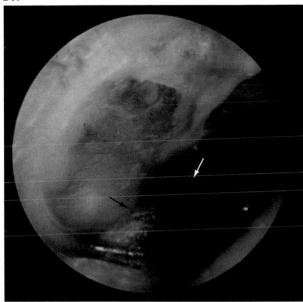

148

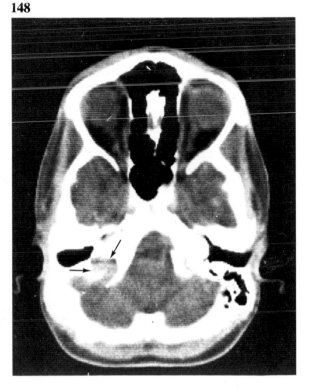

149

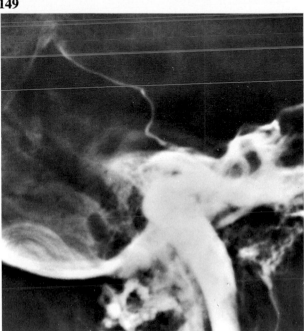

150   High jugular bulb (*see* **150 – 152**) This high
jugular bulb (*arrows*) impinged on the ossicular chain
in this left ear, causing a 30 dB conductive hearing loss.
The patient complained of a 20-year-old history of
tinnitus in this ear. The tinnitus in these patients may be
pulsatile or continuous and may be audible during
auscultation of the patient's ear.

150

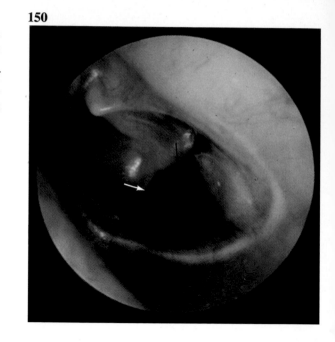

151

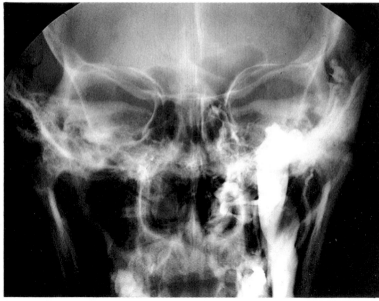

151   High jugular bulb (*see* **150 – 152**) The high
jugular bulb is visualised in the middle ear on this
retrograde jugular venogram (AP view).

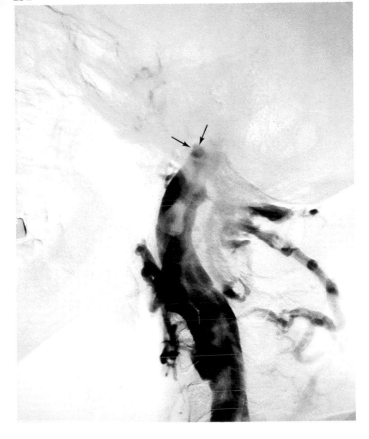

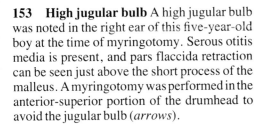

153 High jugular bulb A high jugular bulb was noted in the right ear of this five-year-old boy at the time of myringotomy. Serous otitis media is present, and pars flaccida retraction can be seen just above the short process of the malleus. A myringotomy was performed in the anterior-superior portion of the drumhead to avoid the jugular bulb (*arrows*).

153

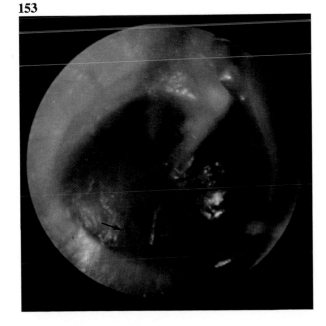

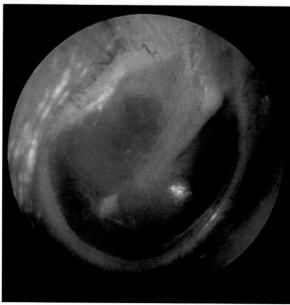

154

Otosclerosis

154 Otosclerosis – Schwartze's sign Otosclerosis is an inherited disease in which a progressive, conductive hearing loss develops, usually in adulthood. The hearing loss is due to fixation of the footplate of the stapes by abnormal bone. In this case, an active otosclerotic focus is faintly visible behind a normal tympanic membrane; the pink blush just to the left of the malleus is termed a Schwartze's sign. The whitish area below the malleus is an old scar. Most patients with otosclerosis have a completely normal otoscopic examination.

155

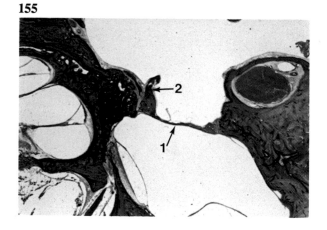

155 Otosclerosis An histological section of a temporal bone of an individual with otosclerosis shows a focus of abnormal bone near the anterior part of the footplate (1) of the stapes (2). This area, the region of the fissula ante fenestrum, is the most common location of otosclerotic foci.

156

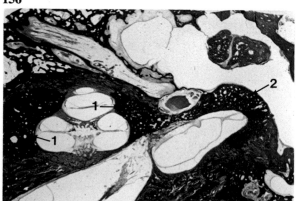

156 Otosclerosis In this histological section, otosclerotic foci are seen as darkly staining portions of vascular bone around the cochlea (1) and the lateral semicircular canal (2). Extensive otosclerosis of this type may lead to sensorineural hearing loss and possibly vertigo.

Trauma

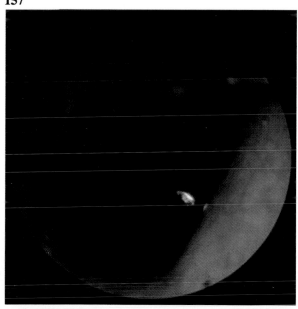

157 Haemotympanum Blood in the middle ear of this patient with a temporal bone fracture gives an almost black appearance to the tympanic membrane.

158 Resolving haemotympanum This patient had sustained a right temporal bone fracture five days previously; the blood in the middle ear has been partially cleared. A few small areas of haematoma remain, but the middle ear contains air.

159 Barotrauma An haemorrhage occurred in the pars flaccida of this right tympanic membrane when this patient sustained barotrauma while scuba diving. The white tympanosclerotic plaques in the pars tensa are unrelated.

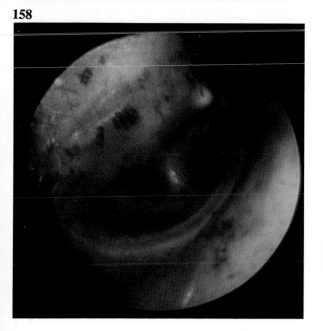

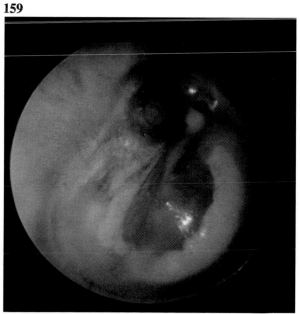

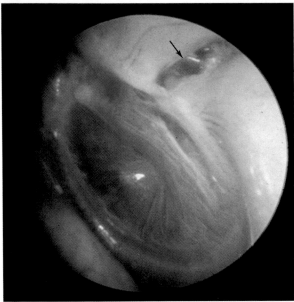

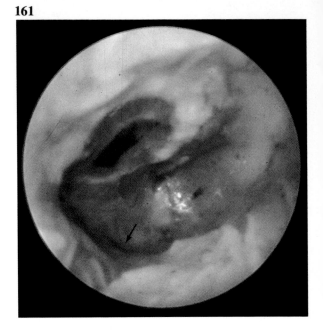

160 Temporal bone fracture Two years after a left, longitudinal temporal bone fracture, this patient had normal hearing. A fracture can be seen extending into the superior auditory canal from the margin of the tympanic membrane (*arrow*). The resultant defect is bridged by an epithelial membrane.

161 Temporal bone fracture Three days after a right, transverse temporal bone fracture, clear cerebrospinal fluid was seen pouring out of this small perforation (*arrow*) in the posterior-superior quadrant of the drumhead. This spinal fluid leak stopped within one week and the perforation healed two weeks later.

162

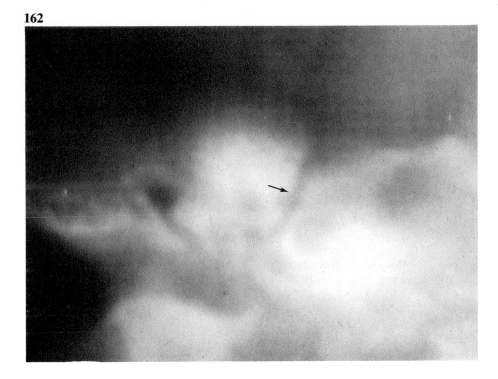

163

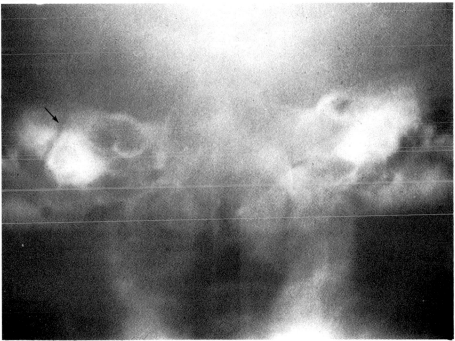

162 & 163 **Temporal bone fracture** Many temporal bone fractures can be confirmed with thin section tomography. These are examples of transverse temporal bone fractures (*arrows*), as seen on coronal section tomography.

164

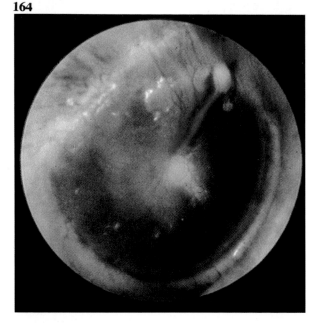

165

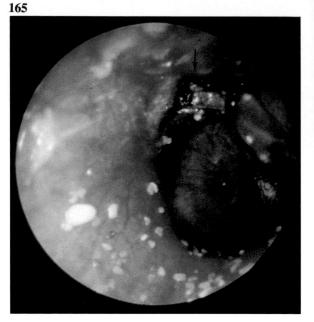

166

164 Barotrauma Sudden decompression while scuba diving led to an haemorrhage in the tympanic membrane and a middle ear effusion in this 20-year-old woman. The haemorrhage is limited, in this case, to the area adjacent to the long process of the malleus.

165 Barotrauma This patient experienced intense pain while scuba diving. Examination of his right ear shows an haemorrhagic area along the annulus of the tympanic membrane. Bleeding from the pars flaccida was observed (*arrow*). Sand is present, adhering to the walls of the external canal wall.

166 Blast trauma An explosion near this patient's right ear resulted in haemorrhages in tympanic membrane and middle ear (*arrows*). This tympanic membrane was retracted and the incus eroded even prior to the blast injury.

Tumours

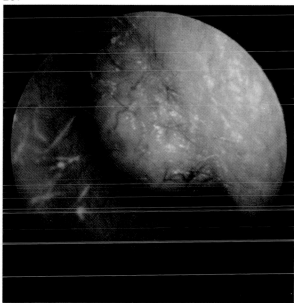

167

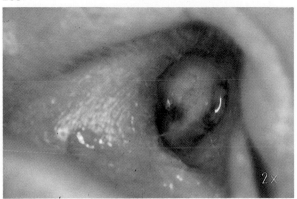

168

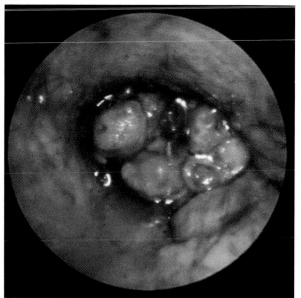

169

167   Benign fibroma This benign fibroma arose from the lateral external auditory canal and caused obstruction of the canal and recurrent external otitis.

168   Squamous carcinoma This is a photograph of the meatus of an ear with a necrotic exophytic tumor arising from the external auditory canal. Carcinomas of the external auditory canal are often misdiagnosed as external otitis and recognised late. In a patient with longstanding external otitis, refractory to medical management, one should consider an underlying carcinoma.

169   Adenocarcinoma This poorly differentiated adenocarcinoma arose from the wall of the external auditory canal. This patient complained of persistent external otitis and severe pain.

170

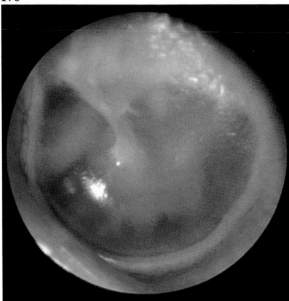

171

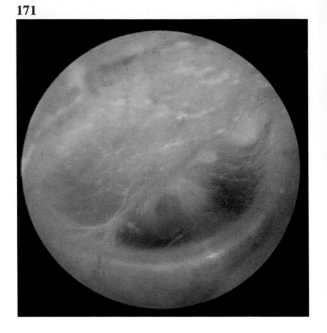

170 Glomus tympanicum This 30-year-old patient had been complaining of pulsatile tinnitus in her left ear for several months. Careful otoscopic evaluation revealed a small red area behind the anterior-inferior quadrant of the tympanic membrane which blanched with air pressure. This represents a glomus tympanicum tumour, which is a benign paraganglioma.

171 Glomus tympanicum This asymptomatic glomus tumour of the middle ear was detected on routine examination. This pulsatile tumour was confined to the middle ear and was removed through a tympanotomy.

Index